365 Days of Health

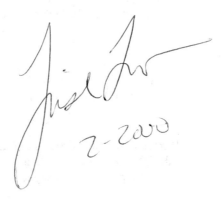

Patricia Telesco

365 Days of Health
A Blue Star Productions
Publication
First Printing: March 1998

ISBN 1-881542-33-5
Copyright © 1998 by Patricia Telesco
An Original Trade Paperback

Published by Blue Star Productions,
A Division of Book World, Inc.
9666 E Riggs Rd. #194
Sun Lakes AZ 85248

Printed in the United States of America
All rights reserved, including the right
of reproduction in any form.

Be sure to visit our web site at:
http://www.bkworld.com

Disclaimer

Neither the author nor the publisher warrant, or make any inferred claim, that the folk traditions presented herein are effective. None of them should be construed as a substitution for proper medical treatment. When conditions persist, please see a doctor, and do not try any remedial to which you might have an allergic reaction. Good health comes from keeping our wits and good judgement keen in the way we take care of our bodies.

Introduction

Health, wealth and happiness — these are the three things for which most people wish. In looking to history, such was the case for our ancestors as well, but for them the health part of this trinity was the most elusive. Lacking the medical knowledge we have today, a person's well being and recuperation often depended on folklore, wive's tales, and familial knowledge.

While many of the folk "prescriptions" seem amusing to the modern mind, they provide unique insight into who we are as a people, and how far we have grown. Then too, laughter is good medicine. One must also remember that many remedies now available in the pharmacy originated in a shaman's, herbalist's, or wise-person's kit. From this perspective we discover even "absurd" approaches sometimes turn out to have merit. For example, who would have ever thought that the use of toad skin to treat heart problems could have actually worked? Yet, toad skin contains a chemical strikingly similar to digitalis!

Gathered into the pages of this book are 365 ways that people have tried to insure themselves of good health or encourage rejuvenation from specific ailments. Rather than repeat the advice you can find readily in home herbals and health guides, this book is dedicated to folk traditions that originated at the hearth and in the heart of so many families around the world. Most of these are perfectly safe to try, if for no other reason than feeling like you're doing something positive to maintain your well being. A positive attitude is, and always has been, at least 60% of the prescription for good health. It speaks to the "mind" that is one third of our whole being (body-mind-spirit).

In the instance where the superstitions are not safe due to toxicities etc., I have provided viable alternatives with which to tinker. In truth, this is sometimes more fun because you can then create a whole new folk custom to share with family and friends. The sharing process allows others to rejoice in your achievement and improve their own health through the revitalizing energy of fellowship. What a tremendous gift that likewise ministers to the spirit!

And what of the body? Well, first remember to be realistic. Folk traditions provide only part of the answer to wholeness. The rest must come by being wise and honoring the temple of our soul. Work, play, and rest each have an important role in maintaining health as does a good diet and regular exercise. Find a balanced combination of these things, adding folk beliefs like icing on the cake, and you will, indeed, live healthier and happier.

Helpful Hints for Using this Book:

You will notice that each day of the year herein is numbered. There are several reasons for this, the primary one of which is flexibility. You do not have to have this book at the beginning of a new year for it to be useful. Instead, use the following chart to discern which day of the year it is, then turn to that part of the book:

January: Day 1-31

February: Day 32-59 (except on a leap

year)
    March: Day 60-90
    April: Day 91-120
    May: Day 121-151
    June: Day 152-181
    July: Day 182-212
    August: Day 213-243
    September: day 244-273
    October: Day 274-304
    November: Day 305-334
    December: Day 335-365

So, say that you receive this book on April 4th as a gift. That equates to 90+4= Day 94. Continue each day forward from here through the year. Mind you, it's ok to peek back and see what you've missed thus far! Additionally, it is perfectly fine, and actually preferable to totally reorganize your approach to health, save those dates that are dependent on a celebration, festival or religious observance.

In reading the entries, sometimes you will notice that animal parts are recommended. This comes from our animistic past wherein humankind revered the animal kingdom for its potent symbolism. In these cases I have included the item as a point of interest, offering some more earth-friendly alternatives. Also, some folk traditions are dependent on timing as a component, specifically the days of the week or phases of the moon. From year to year these days change their format, so if Day 163 talks of a "Monday" action, when it happens to be Wednesday in the current year, simply wait until the next Monday to try the folk tradition.

Most importantly, enjoy this book and have a little fun. Our figurative good health may be found in many things; in seeing the smile of a child, in feeling a spring wind through our hair, or dangling one's feet in cool water on a hot summer day. When one has such blessings in their life somewhat regularly, they indeed may count themselves well and whole.

***

Day 1:

This is the Roman festival honoring Salus, the goddess of health, well being and prosperity. To gain the favor of this Power, simply pray for aid, or leave out an offering of grain.

In Europe children went house-to-house singing, and were then given sausage, onion, chestnuts, apples, sweet cakes, cheese and wine to insure their health, wealth and providence in the New Year.

Day 2:

Wear an eye agate. This keeps illness at bay and protects the bearer from the evil eye.

365 Days of Health

Day 3:

Alsacian tradition recommends cutting one's hair and nails on Friday for improved sight and hearing.

Day 4:

On the third day of the first moon in China, women purify their homes against sickness by carrying steaming vinegar to every room of the house.

Day 5:

Folk tradition dictates that all remedies should be started on a Sunday for increased effectiveness. Sunday was the 7th day of the week, given all the attributes of the Sun and "Son" to empower the remedial.

Day 6:

Have all of your Yule decorations down by now, especially the tree. Not to do so foretells the death of someone in your home.

Day 7:

This is the festival of *Nanakusa* in Japan. It is traditional to eat a rice stew that includes seven different fresh herbs today. This acts as a ward against disease throughout the New Year.

Day 8:

On the 7th day of the first moon in China it is customary to eat red beans for protection against sickness. Women should eat fourteen beans, men should consume seven.

Day 9:

In the Orient, a jade ring is favored for having tremendous curative powers. Put one on when you're feeling out of sorts, or carry a jade stone in your pocket.

Day 10:

During the Carnival at Basel eating brown-flour soup was considered a "sure fire" way of achieving more energy and vitality.

Day 11:

Thought for the day: "All the joys of sense lie in three words: health, peace and competence." -- Alexander Pope.

Day 12:

Nero recommended eating leeks regularly to give yourself a clear voice. For this purpose, they are best planted by the waxing moon. Warm the leek in water and drink for a sore throat.

365 Days of Health

Day 13:

Among Moslems, almonds represent the hope of heaven and the paste is said to have restorative powers (as in Marzipan). In the 16th century a mixture of almonds with diced liver and violet oil was recommended to allay hunger.

Day 14:

Officials at the Carnival in Belgium near Oudenberg once drank wine with gold fish therein, passing the cup around a circle, for health, fertility and abundance.

365 Days of Health

Day 15:

Many wive's tales encourage good eating habits eating as an important component to health. As the old saying goes: "Better the fore part of a horse than the backside of a doctor."

Day 16:

For headaches, bathe your temples in lavender water. Alternatively, wear a sprig of this plant in your hat to avert colds. The scent of lavender prolongs life.

Day 17:

Thought for the day: "There is virtue in the open. There is healing out of doors. The great physician makes his roads along the forest floors." -- Bliss Carman

Day 18:

To cure a fever, gather water from seven different wells (or sinks) and drink thereof. This is an old Spanish remedial.

Day 19:

Saffron simmered in water creates an aroma to dispel sadness, quicken the senses and increase physical energy and alertness. Germans wore this herb as protection against the plague.

Day 20:

Thought for the day: "wine within and oil without is the secret to health and happiness." -- Roman saying.

365 Days of Health

Day 21:

Red coral placed around the neck of a child will protect them from sickness and any trickery of the fairy folk.

Day 22:

Take a piece of cotton or wool string and knot it once for each wart you have. Bury this or toss it in moving water source to carry your warts away.

Day 23:

For curative purposes, 7 knots by 7 knots is thought to be a potent charm. Usually the knots are placed in contact with the problem area then washed in water, buried or burned.

Day 24:

When a child is born, place a lock of its hair at the base of a tree, apple if it is a boy, and peach if it is a girl. The child will then grow as strong and healthy as the tree.

365 Days of Health

Day 25:

Toss a fisherman's net over someone who is ill to ensnare the sickness. This net must then be cast away or burned so no one else gets sick.

Day 26:

Wear an amber necklace to draw out and entrap a sore throat. Or, wear a piece of amber near an inflicted area to draw out pain.

Day 27:

Thought for the day: "There is not joy even in beautiful wisdom unless one have holy health." -- Sextus Empiricus

Day 28:

For headaches the Saxons bind plantain to their forehead with red wool.

Day 29:

Drinking vegetable, beef or chicken broth regularly is believed to purify the body. Using these liquids in a sick room is still quite common, chicken soup being the most popular.

Day 30:

Wear a pouch of salt around your neck and replace the salt every nine days to maintain your health. Or, sprinkle salt around your home to protect everyone therein. Sprinkling salt around a sacred space guards it against negative energy.

365 Days of Health

Day 31:

Wearing a diamond set into a silver ring prevents insomnia, safeguards the wearer from the evil eye and keeps them safe from infectious diseases. Emerald necklaces are reported to have similar effects.

Day 32:

On St. Bride's Eve, placing rushes over your doorway protects the health of all children and animals within the house.

Day 33:

On Candlemas, save a candle from church and keep it lit all the way home. This insures well being, and protects the house and inhabitants from disease.

Day 34:

Invoke St. Blasius today to help protect yourself from throat sicknesses. In Europe, children and pigs alike were given garlic, salt, apples and chocolate for blessings and health.

Day 35:

To rid yourself of corns, rub them with a glove of garlic on Friday during the first quarter of the moon, then throw the clove away.

Day 36:

Thought for the day: "A glass of red wine in an old pot belly is like a new beam in a new bar." -- Old Proverb

Day 37:

For stomachache, dip a comb in holy water then place it in a pot of wine. Lay the come on your stomach for 24 hours, drink one mouthful of the wine, then toss the rest away.

Day 38:

Thought for the day: "Healing is a matter of time, but it is also sometimes a matter of opportunity." -- Hippocrates

365 Days of Health

Day 39:

A mosquito allowed into a sick person's room at sunset will take illness with it when it leaves.

Day 40:

To relieve sore eyes, scrounge nine grains of barley from nine different houses. Make the sign of the cross on each lid with each grain of barley. Toss these behind you and don't look back.

365 Days of Health

Day 41:

To get a lost tooth to grow back, toss the one that fell out into a mouse hole.

Day 42:

Amethyst may be worn or made into a gem elixir to ease headaches, toothache and gout. It protects the wearer from plague, increases one's intellect and stays unruly passions.

Day 43:

Hanging a snake around your neck will relieve fevers or toothaches. This tradition probably has some connection with Hermes' staff bearing two snakes.

Day 44:

On the 8th day of the Chinese New Year people celebrate the birth of humankind. If this date corresponds with the date of your birth (or someone you know) you or that person are guaranteed prosperity, health and joy.

365 Days of Health

Day 45:

A pearl mounted in a pin eases hemorrhages, and banishes jaundice. In powdered form it insures health and prosperity.

Day 46:

In China, this marks the Birthday of the Pearly Emperor. Eating long vermicelli and peaches today bring health and long life.

Day 47:

Thought for the day: "The fool's wisdom comes after he is hurt." -- Japanese Proverb.

Day 48:

Place seven vervain leaves in your walking stick to keep sickness at bay. This type of practice was quite popular in the Victorian Era.

Day 49:

On the 5th day after the birth of a child, carry the baby at a running pace around your hearth (fireplace or stove) with friends and relatives in attendance. This custom comes from Greece where they believed this insured the child of health and sure footedness.

Day 50:

To preserve one's eyesight, wear a gold ring in your left ear and wash both eyes in the water from a sacred fountain. If you don't wear earrings, try any gold piece of jewelry like a tie tack or ring.

Day 51:

For a fever repeat the following incantation seven times: "red dragon, white dragon, blue dragon fly! I conjure you to go in the eye of the fattest toad you can find!"

Day 52:

Light all the lamps in your house today and any candles you can find until the morrow. Traditionally this was the Feast of Lights in China where each light represents the fire of the soul. For the living this insures longevity; for the dead it acts as a prayer of peace.

Day 53:

Placing bay laurel in your doorways will protect everyone who enters your home from sickness.

Day 54:

In Armenia people surround themselves with pieces of iron to avert the spirit of disease called *al*. This is particularly protective for child bearing women.

Day 55:

Thought for the day: "After dinner rest a while, after supper walk a mile." -- Old Proverb.

Day 56:

The Greeks bound olive leaves with the name of Athena written upon them around their forehead to cure headaches. The writing of the name of this goddess upon the leaf was a type of invocation for aid.

Day 57:

Wear turquoise as a talisman to warn when your health is in danger. Should you become ill, its color will fade or the stone will shatter.

Day 58:

To create a potion that protects you from all illness, gather 4 rue branches at noon along with 9 juniper berries, a walnut, a dried fig and a pinch of salt. Steep these for 9 hours in water then consume on an empty stomach.

365 Days of Health

Day 59:

Thought for the day: "Some patients recover their health simply through their contentment with the goodness of the physician." -- Hippocrates

Day 60:

In Newfoundland an infusion of alder buds is recommended for itching, and a salve from the bark for minor applying to burns.

365 Days of Health

Day 61:

Today is a sacred day for Ceadda, a spirit of healing springs and holy wells. Bathe in flower water today for well being.

Day 62:

The Shoshone Indians carry powdered spruce needles to prevent illness. Hopi Indians similarly use petrified wood.

Day 63:

A Talmudic spell against blindness is to say "my mother hath warned be to beware of shabriri, abriri, riri, ri!" This makes the demon of blindness shrink with his name.

Day 64:

Passing yourself under a bramble bush will gather burns or flu into the tangles, and leave you well.

Day 65:

Ivory bracelets, amulets or other forms of jewelry protect the wearer from sickness, especially cancer. To be most effective the ivory should be boiled in sea water with mandrake root before being fashioned.

Day 66:

Indian folklore recommends wearing a red thread around one's neck to protect them from *acheri*, the female spirit of sickness. Alternatively, wear a red scarf or shirt.

Day 67:

Place a clean quartz crystal in spring water and let it steep for three hours by the light of a waning moon. Take the stone out and drink the liquid so sickness may shrink. Alternatively, place it in the light of a waxing to full moon so physical energy increases.

Day 68:

Thought for the day: "Good health and good sense are two of life's greatest blessings." -- Publilius Syrus

Day 69:

During Siamese New Year people traditionally wear an unspun cotton cord around the shoulders to expel all negativity and sickness. Alternatively, wear a cotton shirt skirt, or other piece of clothing.

Day 70:

In Greece people believed they could be healed, or learn of a source of healing, through divinely inspired dreams. For this you must bathe and fast, then go to a holy temple or church and sleep the night in the sanctum.

365 Days of Health

Day 71:

To rid yourself of pain for one day eat 4 sprigs of rue along with a fig, a nut, a pinch of salt and 9 juniper berries.

Day 72:

To cure a fever, drive a nail into the trunk of a tree. This attaches the fever to the tree, which then "grounds out" the illness.

Day 73:

For vigor and health, pass over the hollow cavity in an oak tree nine times.

Day 74:

Palm Sunday (est. date 3/15-4/18) was once known as "box day" as people customarily placed blessed box tree branches in their homes, above the bed and in the barn. This was considered an effective protection from illness and demons.

Day 75:

This is the Holi festival in India. For overcoming winter illnesses, toss a cake of what flour and chick peas into a fire source..

Day 76:

This is the festival of Liber in Greece. Youths take their first draughts of wine today for health and longevity. Note: grape juice will suffice.

Day 77:

Between the second and third moon of the year, the Chinese celebrate a festival of cold foods called *Han Shih* . On this day all fires are extinguished in honor of Kwan Yin, a compassionate goddess, and cold food is eaten for health.

Day 78:

On St. Joseph's Day in Italy people consume lentil soup and long noodles for long life, and leafy vegetables for providence and prosperity.

Day 79:

Thought for the day: "Medicine, to produce health, has to examine disease just as music, to create harmony, must investigate discord." -- Plutarch.

Day 80:

An Arabian talisman for good blood is wearing an arrow fashioned from agate as a necklace or other portable charm.

Day 81:

Children should wear blue in infancy to guard them from all sickness. Alternatively, paint their room blue instead.

Day 82:

The French eat spinach greens on Maundy Thursday at lunch time to avoid stomach ailments throughout the year. Additionally, a loaf of round bread hung from the ceiling will ward off disease today.

On Maundy Thursday in the Pennsylvania Dutch tradition, one should eat green vegetables for health.

Day 83:

An egg laid on Good Friday, when kept on the mantle, wards off the spirit of sickness and facilitates teething in children. Additionally, blowing through the key hole of a church today before sunrise is a charm against urinary disorders, and any water dipped before sunrise in silence has healing powers.

Day 84:

In ancient Rome this was the festival of Hilaria when laughing was believed to be a healthful activity. See a good comedy or tell some jokes today!

Day 85:

To maintain your health, never sleep in the moonlight. This is considered physically bad and may cause lunacy.

Day 86:

In Egypt this is Smell the Breeze day when taking walks and enjoying the fresh air is believed to have tremendous healthful outcomes. Try going for a good long stroll in the park today.

Day 87:

Thought for the day: "Joy, temperance and repose slam the door on the Doctor's nose." -- Longfellow

Day 88:

Press the roof of your mouth with your thumb to ease a headache.

365 Days of Health

Day 89:

Knots were often used by healers to bind various ailments. For this to work, the cord should be a sympathetic color to the problem, for example using yellow for jaundice, and red for blood ailments. Next the rope or string needs to be laid against the inflicted area and knotted 7 or 9 times, each time saying "I bind this _____ (fill in appropriately). Then the rope or string should be tossed into running water to carry away the malady.

Day 90:

Early in the spring eat a daisy to avert summer fevers. This should be done on an empty stomach. An alternative is eating 9 leaves from the first stalk of wheat you find later in the season.

Day 91:

Take a piece of cotton or wool string and knot it once for each wart you have. Bury this or toss it in moving water source to carry your warts away.

Day 92:

In Italy, garlic in the pantry protects the home from sickness, especially those caused by foods. Try suspending whole garlic in olive oil and use this in cooking, too.

Day 93:

Make yourself a bath with rue, sorrel and thyme floating therein. This aids recuperation and helps protect you from future contagion.

Day 94:

Some folk remedials recommend burying a person in soil, mud or sand up to their head to allay sickness. Effectively this is a mock death that fools the spirit of the illness into leaving, which is then entrapped in the earth.

Day 95:

Onions placed in a sick room will attract germs and help quicken recovery. This tradition comes from Britain.

Day 96:

Break a newly laid egg over an ant hill to break a fever.

Day 97:

To know if a sick person is soon to recover, the Potawatum plains Indians take the inner seed from a Jack-in-the-Pulpit and drop it in a cup of water. If it circles the cup four times clockwise before it sinks, recovery is imminent.

Day 98:

"To live long, keep a cool head and warm feet. -- Japanese proverb

365 Days of Health

Day 99:

Wrap copper wire around your wrist or waist to ease the pain in sore joints. This custom is found both in early America and Africa.

Day 100:

Carrying a buckeye (horse chestnut) is a talisman against pain. An alternative is carrying a new potato until it turns black and gets hard. It must then be replaced.

365 Days of Health

Day 101:

Wearing a red flannel scarf around your neck prevents nose bleeds.

Day 102:

For a stitch in your side, stop long enough to pick up a stone and spit upon it. Place the stone exactly back where it laid, with the wet side down and the pain will abate.

Day 103:

Tie a string around the small toe of your right foot to combat a toothache.

Day 104:

To protect everyone in your home from colds and sore throats, place a plumb branch in the fire place.

Day 105:

Thought for the day: "An hour's sleep before midnight is worth three after." -- Old Proverb

Day 106:

Stand on your head and take a spoonful of sugar to cure hiccups. Or, hold your nose and swallow nine times.

Day 107:

To know if your food or drink has any harmful impurities, serve it from a jade plate or cup. In the Orient, people believe that jade is so pure that it will crack if touched by any poisons.

Day 108:

The Welsh wash a diseased area with a rag, then take that rag to a nearby tree to transfer the illness to the bower. In the interest of ecology, use only a small natural fiber piece.

Day 109:

Thought for the day: "Be sober and temperate and you will be healthy." -- Benjamin Franklin.

Day 110:

Those who suffer from joint problems should wear a buzzard's feather behind their ear.

Day 111:

Parilia in Rome. Drinking milk mixed with must, sprinkling yourself with sacred waters, and sweeping the house with a bay broom will protect your health.

Day 112:

Open a pair of scissors to form a cross and hide it in a pillow or drawer to protect against illnesses.

Day 113:

To keep a splinter from getting infected blow on it 9 times and place two pieces of linen that form a cross thereon while invoking the blessing of St. Como and St. Damien, both noted for their healing arts.

Day 114:

Keep pimpernel in your home. It protects everyone within the house from sickness and accidents.

Day 115:

Sacrament monies carried around the communion table three times averts joint problems if worn on a chain regularly.

Day 116:

In Cornwall, passing through a large holed rock, or a tree split in two, cures sickness by marking the transition into health.

Day 117:

Thought for the day: "If you want to know if your brain is flabby, feel your legs." -- Bruce Barton

Day 118:

Late in April the Feast of *Gula* was celebrated in Babylonia, honoring this goddess of healing and life preservation. To encourage the presence of this Power, place images or statues of dogs around your home.

Day 119:

On the celtic calendar this marks the beginning of the runic month of Flowing Water (*lagu*). Take a long, restful bath and visualize your tensions moving down the drain!

Day 120:

Ashes from Walpurgis night/Beltane Eve may be scattered on the land or in one's home to protect against any literal or figurative blights.

Day 121:

Dew gathered on May 1 before sunrise, and applied to the skin, gives beauty and treats skin conditions. In China this dew is regarded as a panacea that renews life in the dying.

Day 122:

Folk traditions tell us to never pay the doctor's bill in full, or you will grow sick again.

Day 123:

Wearing a crab shell promotes well being and protects the bearer from malevolent magic.

Day 124:

Ascension day is 40 days after Easter. Germans gather medicinal herbs today believing them to be more potent. Italians believe that miraculous cures can be performed at the stroke of midnight beginning this festival, and some people hang red and white wreaths over their doors to protect the occupants of the house from all calamities.

Day 125:

The *Tango no sekku* festival in Japan. Flying carp banners and kites near your home today brings strength and vigor to all male children within, and dolls of mugwort hung off the gates of your home will dispel all negative aires.

Day 126:

Gather anemone blossoms in the spring and wrap them in red cloth. When carried this bundle promotes health and protects the bearer from disease.

Day 127:

The gourd-like fruit of the Calabash tree may be used in making pictoral charms for wellness, but the tree must be planted on St. John's Day to be truly effective.

Day 128:

Thought for the day: "Elevate the desire for health, youth and longevity to the position of a religion." -- Rabbi Wise

365 Days of Health

Day 129:

To clear up warts, touch each with a green pea than toss over your left shoulder and don't look back.

Day 130:

Lie on some freshly dug earth and breath into a hole for one quarter hour to rid yourself of a cold. Effectively, the symbolism here is breathing the cold into the soil.

Day 131:

Arabians carry yellow coral, or tie pieces to a tree, for strength and long life. If this ever breaks, you need to get a new coral amulet as the breakage releases the magic.

Day 132:

Plant a window box with rosemary seeds. The smell increases physical energy and youthfulness.

Day 133:

To rid yourself of corns, steep a pearl in lemon juice until its dissolved. Apply this by soaking a slice of lemon in the mixture and placing this on the corn never day until it can easily be extracted. This tradition comes from England.

365 Days of Health

Day 134:

For protection or relief from migraines, wear a crown of braided ivy mingled with cabbage leaves.

Day 135:

During flu season place four ferns with chicory root in four cups of boiling water. Add one spoonful of honey and stir clockwise with a licorice stick. Drink this between meals.

Day 136:

Thought for the day: "Some people think that doctors and nurses can put scrambled eggs back into the shell." -- Dorothy Canfield

Day 137:

To fight weariness, place mugwoart in your shoes and take a tea of it before going to bed at night. This herb is also believed to counteract sunstroke symptoms.

Day 138:

If you want to be sure your physician makes the right diagnosis of a problem, give him or her a green jasper. The physicians of the Middle Ages often wore this stone as an amulet for similar purposes.

Day 139:

English legend claims that three balm leaves placed in a cup of beer and consumed four times over twelve days provides recovery by the 12th day.

Day 140:

Hopi Indians recommend juniper greens boiled in water to ease a sour stomach and eliminate constipation. They use the berries to combat colds and colic in children.

Day 141:

Nine grains of wheat rubbed on a boil and tossed into a fire makes the boil disappear.

Day 142:

The Cat's eye or Tiger's eye was a favorite ancient talisman for protection from eye problems. Additionally, the Assyrians believed this granted invisibility from one's enemies, and in China people wore the stone to combat asthma and improve facial color.

365 Days of Health

Day 143:

To protect yourself from nose bleeds, wear a key on a chain and allow it to dangle down the back of your neck.

Day 144:

This marks the Festival of Hermes Trismegistus, the patron of Alchemy and Medicine whose emblem is the caduceus. An excellent day to schedule a physical with your doctor.

Day 145:

Headaches caused by over exposure to heat should be treated by placing a ball of lax on a yellow plate and balancing it on your head for seven minutes. Burn the flax afterwards. This is an Italian tradition.

Day 146:

In Germany roast camomile was brewed in vinegar and used as a mouth wash. Dabbing this on a toothache also eases the pain.

365 Days of Health

Day 147:

Thought for the day: "Precautions must be taken <u>first</u>." -- Japanese Proverb

Day 148:

Basil was a sacred herb in many cultures. Galen recommended it for emotional well being. In India, it is grown in pots near the home to protect every part of the body.

Day 149:

In Ireland, drinking holy water from a silver bell is believed to drive away the spirit of sickness. One caution, make sure that the silver hasn't recently been polished.

Day 150:

Sit for three hours with your back against an oak tree to make your backache go away. This is also a very effective way to ground unwanted or excess energy.

Day 151:

The Feast of Corpus Cristi in France takes place around this time of year (between 5/21 and 6/24). Anyone who can pass between the cross and the processional banners today will be protected from colds for the year.

Day 152:

The Festival of Carna in ancient Rome where the goddess who presides over matters of physical health is offered beans and bacon. You might wish to make a similar dish, placing a little outside as your offering and consuming the rest.

Day 153:

In the Middle east, offering an agate to god in June brings health and eloquence to the worshiper. The green and red version of this stone was considered an antidote for poison, and the white agate will keep one's eyes clear if carried as an amulet.

365 Days of Health

Day 154:

In Ireland bracken tea is applied to burns and scalds to ease pain.

Day 155:

Sacred writings on parchment or in a small book, when carried, become a talisman for health. The verses chosen should have something to do with maintaining well-being or recovery.

Day 156:

Lodestone bound to the bottom of your feet draws out illness and preserves virility. Additionally, if mounted in gold it strengthens the heart.

Day 157:

Thought for the day: "Amusement is a commodity essential to physical and mental health and well being." -- Milton Sills

Day 158:

Gather club moss on the third day of the moon with clean hands while saying "do what thou cuttest, cuttest for good." Boil this in spring water and apply it to swellings.

Day 159:

In England and Teutonic regions drinking mead (honey wine) was believed to preserve health, most likely due to the cooking process used which made the beverage safer than water.

Day 160:

During the spring make yourself a tonic from daisy petals for health, devotion and love. Steep the daisies in warm water to create a tea and sweeten to taste.

Day 161:

For aches and sores on the skin Shinnecock Indians warm kelp and apply it directly.

Day 162:

The best time to prepare herbal medicines and healthful tonics is when the mon is first beginning to be revealed after an eclipse.

Day 163:

Take a cloth figurine (poppet) and stuff it with any healthful herbs like garlic buds, lemon balm, eucalyptus, etc. Sew it shut and keep it in a safe place to encourage well being. When the poppet looses its aroma, burn it and make a new one.

Day 164:

In Italy, children are given flint to safeguard their well-being. In Burma this stone is said to prevent appendicitis, and Japan it is worn as a charm against ulcers.

Day 165:

Set up an archway made from dogwood limbs and pass though it. Burn the limbs afterward to burn away any germs.

Day 166:

Hang an egg around your neck for seven or nine days to collect any illness in your body, then bury the egg. Alternatively, rub it on the afflicted area, then break it open into the garbage.

Day 167:

On, or around, this date in Egypt the Nile begins to rise. Put a lump of clay outside your door at dusk. If it is cracked by morning, it symbolizes a long, healthy life.

Day 168:

In Morocco a person wishing to improve their fertility would gather seven keys from seven houses in seven towns and heat them until red hot. These were then cooled with water and the person exposed themselves to the steam.

Day 169:

Thought for the day: "He who has health, has hope. He who has hope has everything." -- Arabic proverb.

365 Days of Health

Day 170:

Dig up a fern root when the sun is in Leo and hit it somewhere in your bedroom to prevent tooth decay. Save the leaves from the plant for Day 211.

Day 171:

During midsummer festivals, jumping over the flames or passing through the smoke thereto is a way to purify and protect yourself from sickness. This is also true of Beltane (Day 121). Please make sure, however, that the fires a low and well tended for safety.

Day 172:

In Morocco, people diving into any flowing water source during midsummer festivals to cleans and protect themselves from sickness. They also do this for their animals.

Day 173:

Midsummer's eve is the best time to harvest herbs that are going to be used in magical folk remedies. This increases their power, but take care not to cut them with any iron implement or the magic is lost.

Day 174:

On St. John's eve, gather a four leaf clover at midnight. Carried on your person this draws health, love, fortune and fame to you.

Day 175:

On St. John's day, wear walnut leaves to improve blood circulation. Italians gather sap from the sacred oak tree to heal wounds. Russians use today's dew to remove freckles and eye ailments. Finally, balancing a child over a St. John's fire 9 times will give them physical strength and courage.

Day 176:

In Germany people look through larkspur branches toward the midsummer fires to keep their eyes clear and healthy for another year.

Day 177:

"The best physic is to preserver health." -- Francis Bacon

Day 178:

To make a medicine bundle that encourages health, place vervain, dill, rowan, juniper, flax, holly, and a clove of garlic in a red felt bag and carry it with you regularly.

Day 179:

Thought for the day: "Eat an apple before going to bed, make the Doctor beg for bread." -- Old Proverb.

Day 180:

In Italy, an arrow shaped pendant is considered effective protection from the spirit of illness. In Arabia similar pendants are worn to help blood problems and in France they facility safe childbirth.

Day 181:

In the Lusi shrine of Artemis, a well known healing center, the herb artemisia was ignited by a torch for health. If you can't find artemisia, use sage instead.

Day 182:

During the summer months to ease the discomfort caused by insect bites prepare a solution of vinegar, onion juice, garlic juice and lemon juice. Rub this into the bite and blow upon it. This really works.

Day 183:

Ginseng in China is the ultimate tonic that cures all ills, perfecting health, vigor, and even extending life. It may be consumed in tea or wine.

Day 184:

Asafetida gum resin mixed with grave dirt, ashes and nail parings is a West Indian amulet to protect the bearer from disease.

Day 185:

To purify your body, wash yourself in ashes from a Sacred fire (India). Similar customs exist in France for swellings, in Bosnia for skin eruptions and in Morocco to keep hair from falling out.

Day 186:

The Pueblo Indians recite medicinal formulas in reverse order to encourage an illness to likewise reverse itself.

365 Days of Health

Day 187:

"The wise for cure on exercise depend." -- John Dryden

Day 188:

During an eclipse, turn all your pots and dishes upside down (Yukon Indians) to turn away any ill influences. Also, eat no fruit gathered during the eclipse as this it is not healthy (Swabian).

Day 189:

Eat one cypress seed each day. The Greeks felt this would make you strong, healthy, youthful, and sharpen the senses.

Day 190:

Decorate one object in your home with a diamond (a herkimer diamond will suffice). In India people believe this insures longevity, beauty, vitality and joy. Another stone that may be substituted is quartz.

Day 191:

Thought for the day: "Early to bed, early to rise, makes a man healthy, wealthy and wise." -- Old Proverb.

Day 192:

To encourage the health of those you love, greet them tenderly. As a Spanish proverb tells us "hugs and kisses do not break bones."

Day 193:

Save the umbilical cord from a new born and give it to them when they become adults. This is considered a powerful amulet for health, and is featured in many folk remedials.

Day 194:

In a small pouch place a little camphor, caraway, coriander, figwort, galangal, juniper, and marjoram. Wear this around your neck to keep you safe from colds and flu.

Day 195:

In the celtic calendar this marks the beginning of the *ur* cycle, devoted to strength. Eat foods noted for their positive virility like spinach.

Day 196:

Pots of red geraniums in and around your home encourage strength and health. In Mexico these flowers were used to brush patients thereby purifying them.

Day 197:

On the 15th day of the 7th moon in China, the Ancestors are propitiated with burnt paper images of all good things in life. The people believe if this is not done, the spirits will inhabit the grass and bring plagues.

Day 198:

"Don't call the doctor *after* the funeral." -- Japanese Proverb.

Day 199:

In Scotland pilgrimages to sacred wells are made during this time of year. Each person carries a piece of tin cut to represent any inflicted body part. This is hung on a near by tree with a ribbon while prayers are said to St. Thenew, a great healer. An option for your own home might be making a wind chime similarly, and placing it in any tree near your home to ring in wellness.

365 Days of Health

Day 200:

All folk remedials should be repeated thrice or 3 times 3 to be effective.

Day 201:

Letting a chain drag behind your vehicle protects the owner from heartburn and bellyaches. This is partly where the custom of dragging shoes behind a newlywed's car began.

Day 202:

The word Abracadabra, which translates to mean "perish like the word", when written in descending form and worn around the neck is a charm for inflammations:

ABRACADABRA
ABRACADABR
ABRACADAB
ABRACADA
ABRACAD
ABRACA
ABRAC
ABRA
ABR
AB
A

After wearing the charm for seven days toss it into running water that is moving away from you.

Day 203:

Wear or carry red stones if you have blood problems, particularly with your circulation. This idea comes from the Law of Similars in folk medicine where like cures like (red being the color of blood).

365 Days of Health

Day 204:

Put a house leek on your roof to protect the entire family from infection.

Day 205:

Garlic is an age-old protector from sickness and considered an effective tonic even for one's pets. The odor scares off the spirits of disease.

Day 206:

Wheat grains blessed by a holy person are an effective ward against colds and flu. Tossed over the shoulder these can also get rid of warts.

Day 207:

In Brittany July 26-27 is St. Anne's Festival. To cure any illness, and bring favorable outcomes in trials, one should leave the Saint a votive offering today.

Day 208:

"A sound mind in a sound body; if the former be the glory of the latter, the latter is indispensable to the former." -- Tryon Edwards

Day 209:

"Sickness and sorrows come and go, but a superstitious soul hath no rest." -- Robert Burton 1621

Day 210:

Roses have numerous folk remedial applications including in a tea as a tonic with high vitamin C, and applied to the skin in compress form. However, you should always ask permission of the plant before picking it and leave some type of gift in compensation for the petals.

Day 211:

Burn the fern leave from Day 170 for protection against inset bites and any pestilence they carry. Traditionally this is part of the Feast of St. Abdon, the patron of hygiene.

Day 212:

The beginning of the Celtic cycle of defense (*Thorn*). Take extra care with getting proper vitamins into your system.

Day 213:

On Lammas in Scotland some people sprinkle milk on the doorways to safeguard the household from sickness through the fall and winter. Originally this threshold sacrifice was cow's blood.

Day 214:

In ancient Macedonia today was a festival honoring the Dryads, the spirits who inhabit the woods or water sources. To safeguard yourself from infliction today, if you must do any washing carry iron or a nail with you.

Day 215:

"Regimen is better than physic. Everyone should be his own physician. We out to assist and not force nature." -- Voltaire

Day 216:

A remedy for fevers in New England instructs that one bandage burdock leaves point down on the wrist and ankle so that the fever will follow the direction of the leaf, out of the body.

Day 217:

Jumping over a new grave takes away disease and overcomes death. Please take care to honor the sacredness of the region.

Day 218:

"A wise physician recognizes that his only mission is to prepare the way for one greater than himself — nature." -- A.S. Hardy

Day 219:

The Tao cross (ankh) of the Egyptians literally symbolizes the breath or key of life. Wear it as a restorative, generative emblem.

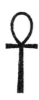

Day 220:

Carry jade to deter kidney and bladder problems. This is an Eastern tradition.

Day 221:

Interesting fact: The prophet Mohammed believed salt had properties that helped overcome 70 diseases.

Day 222:

Place coral, a fresh mint sprig, orange rind, and apple peel in a green or red cloth and tie it up with a white thread. Carry this to encourage health.

Day 223:

Rainwater is considered an effective treatment to eye illness simply by rinsing the eyes with it.

Day 224:

In Armenia, no grapes are allowed to be harvested until this date, at which time they are blessed, then consumed in many dishes for continued abundance and health.

Day 225:

Hang basil in and around your home to take away all eye ailments and purify the air for healthier living quarters.

Day 226:

Fashion a belt from fern leaves and wear it. This cures all illness.

Day 227:

On the 15th day of the 8th moon is the festival of the Moon in china. Today people eat moon shaped cakes and watermelon cut in the shape of a lotus for continued well being. Some of this food may be offered to the Moon to encourage favor.

Day 228:

Between now and August 28th, pilgrimages take place to the healing waters of Lourdes. This is a good time of year to join a health spa, or go to a hot tub for relaxation.

Day 229:

Thought for the day: "Half the spiritual difficulties that men and women suffer arise from a morbid state of health." -- H.W. Beecher

Day 230:

Wear 13 cloves of garlic for 13 days then throw the bundle over your shoulder at a cross road. Don't turn back and your sickness will stay with the garlic.

365 Days of Health

Day 231:

To get a cinder out of your eye, rub the other or blow out of the opposite side of your nose.

365 Days of Health

Day 232:

To relieve a sprain apply to rings of braided reed to the twist and bathe the area in an unguent of red wine and honey.

Day 233:

Take the wash water from a sick room and toss it on a stray animal. They will then run off with the illness on their heels.

Day 234:

Cork placed between the sheets or held in the hand for three nights then buried will absorb sickness.

Day 235:

During the Middle Ages, sage was considered a cure all. Gather it with our right hand and leave bread and wine for the plant, then carry it as an amulet for health and wisdom.

Day 236:

The smoke from burning juniper wood dispels infection. The oil from this tree also aids back aches when rubbed into the skin.

365 Days of Health

Day 237:

For blisters, apply a poultice of beech leaves. For chapped lips and painful gums, chew the leaves instead.

Day 238:

If you have any friends that are under the weather, this is the traditional day in Breton to intercede on their behalf with St. Anne.

Day 239:

"Health is the soul that animates all the enjoyments of life, which fade and are tasteless without it." -- Sir W. Temple

Day 240:

Wrap your foods in lotus petals when serving. This insures the meal will benefit your body.

Day 241:

Nine star stones (small quartz crystals) gathered form a running brook and boiled in the same water give restorative qualities to the water. This is a British superstition.

Day 242:

To keep germs out of your house, string onions across the doorway. This was common in old New England.

Day 243:

In North West India, the first sheath of grain that is reaped is mixed with milk and sugar then consumed to insure the whole family of health and sweetness.

Day 244:

Among the ancient Hebrews a very ill person might change their name to that of an inanimate, ugly object to fool the spirit of sickness into leaving.

365 Days of Health

Day 245:

Drink an infusion of life-everlasting once daily for health and longevity.

Day 246:

Eating three lark eggs on Sunday before the bells ring will bring recuperation from any malady. I suggested regular eggs cooked instead for safety.

Day 247:

Place horehound leaves in the room of a sick person to promote recovery and continuing protection.

Day 248:

"He lives well who knows what is enough." -- Japanese Proverb

365 Days of Health

Day 249:

Mexicans celebrate a holiday honoring the Virgin of the Remedies with dance and incense today in traditional Aztec fashion to encourage continued health.

Day 250:

In the Himalayan region, today marks the festival of Durga. Effigies get burned today, and the ashes are taken home as cures for any eye problems over the next year.

Day 251:

On the 9th day of the 9th moon, people in china drink a wine made from Aster stems and leaves for longevity and health.

Day 252:

The Chrysanthemum festival in Japan. Add these flowers to a salad today, or steep them in wine to increase your longevity.

Day 253:

Thought for the day: "A pale cobbler is better than a sick king." -- Issac Bickerstaff

Day 254:

For stress related maladies, make lettuce tea and drink of it. Also wash your brow with the tincture.

Day 255:

Take a daily tonic of lavender, rose, fennel, cinnamon, and caraway tea at sunrise and sunset to safeguard your health.

365 Days of Health

Day 256:

For protection against cancer, drink nettle, lily and mulberry tea once a month.

Day 257:

Thought for the day: "The physical is the substratum of the spiritual." -- William Tyndale

Day 258:

This is the Birthday of the Moon in China when all foods of the harvest are taken to rooftops to bask in the moonlight so their nutritional value increases.

Day 259:

To improve your sleep, try a tincture of rose, myrtle, Valarian, and vervain.

Day 260:

To break a cold and fever, take ten drops of white vinegar steeped with cloves for three days.

Day 261:

When you must go to a healer try to find one whose parents had the same surname, or the 7th son of a 7th son. Both individuals in Ireland are thought to have improved healing powers.

365 Days of Health

Day 262:

If your child has a cow lick, this indicates they will be healthy and intelligent.

365 Days of Health

Day 263:

The Birthday of the Sun in Peru. Greet the morning sunrays with a cup of wine. Pour half of this out as an offering to the sun, and give the rest to yourself and your family in a gold cup for health.

365 Days of Health

Day 264:

The Irish believe that if you can find just the right hair on the back of the head and pull it out, this will alleviate headaches and head colds forever.

Day 265:

Wash your face in sun touched dew each morning for health and creativity. This also enhances inner beauty.

Day 266:

Always make your doctor's appointments on Thursday, the most propitious time for healing.

Day 267:

"To preserve health is a moral and religious duty; for health is the basis of all social virtues." -- Samuel Johnson

Day 268:

The water used to cool forged iron is said to have healing properties.

Day 269:

In Africa, fever caused by infection from a cut may be cured by keeping the tool cool. This illustrates the Law of Sympathy where treating the tool likewise treats the patient.

Day 270:

Catch a falling oak leaf before it hits the ground and you will be free of colds throughout the fall and winter. This tradition originates in England and Germany.

Day 271:

An old remedy for dysentery recommends mixing a raw egg yoke in brandy and drinking this beverage. Just take care that the egg is fresh.

Day 272:

To maintain health and avoid liver problems, take a glass of red wine with a gold coin there in and place it under the stars for three nights. Put this mixture in a smaller glass and drink it in equal portions over the next three days at the first sign of dawn.

Day 273:

The Romans made offerings to Medetrina today, the goddess of medicine. Another good day for a checkup. Alternatively, leave a candle and rose petals out as a prayer to St. Theresa for intercession in health matters.

Day 274:

Vervain root dung under a waning moon and cut in two pieces may be used to banish illness. One half is placed around the patient's neck, and the other in a dish over a fire. When the fired half is dried completely by the flames the problem will abate.

Day 275:

To keep your eyes keen, anoint the lids daily with honey (carefully please). An alternate might be eating honey glazed carrots.

Day 276:

Moroccan New Year. Take the ashes from any straw fire and wrap them in calico as a charm for good health. Also wash yourself with water at dawn to keep sickness away.

Day 277:

"Never hurry, take plenty of exercise; always be cheerful and take all the sleep you need, and you may expect to be well."
-- J.P. Clarke

Day 278:

For swelling, mix warm oatmeal with oil of roses and apply to the afflicted area.

Day 279:

To keep yourself well, mix 3 handfuls of soil from three mole hills with vinegar and place this mixture in three equally spaced spots around your home.

Day 280:

To get rid of moles, pimples or warts, rub a bean against each saying "as this bean shall rot away so my _____ (wart/mole) shall soon decay." Bury the bean beneath an ash tree.

365 Days of Health

Day 281:

To treat a burn or scald using folk magic, repeat the verbal charm "out fire, in frost" while inscribing a sacred symbol over the region nine times.

Day 282:

"For every evil under the sun, there is a remedy or there is none! If there be one, try to find it; if there be none, never mind it! -- Folk Saying

Day 283:

Hindus recommend looking at an emerald to improve one's appetite and relieve eye strain.

365 Days of Health

Day 284:

In Holland, people carry stale bread or put a piece in a baby's cradle as protection against disease. Egyptians lick the bread instead to cure indigestion.

365 Days of Health

Day 285:

In ancient Egypt the eye of Horus was worn as an amulet to encourage well being:

Eye of Horus

Day 286:

A dragon image carved on a red stone brings health and joy to the bearer. Alternatively a ram carved in sapphire protects against and cures all illness.

365 Days of Health

Day 287:

If you find a brown feather it portends health. A black and white one signifies averting all physical difficulty.

Day 288:

"The first wealth is health." -- Ralph Waldo Emerson

Day 289:

The astrological sign of centaurus was once used as a magical sigil for maintaining health and fertility.

Day 290:

Wear cat's eye on Thursday to protect yourself from all sickness.

Day 291:

If you dream of bathing this foretells long life and vitality. Dreaming of jade or coral is an omen of restored health.

Day 292:

For pain or swelling use a poultice of powdered coral with ash leaves touched upon the troubled area. Bury this under an old oak tree to bury the problem.

Day 293:

Braid three strands of red wool and wear this on your wrist to prevent arthritis. Or, put the wool near to the malady (like around your ankle for a foot problem).

Day 294:

Mix dandelion, marigolds, and tobacco leaves in warm water and apply them to insect bites or stings for relief.

Day 295:

When you have a cold, keep seven beans in your pocket. Toss one away each day, after which time you should be well.

Day 296:

To keep your eyesight keen, rinse your eyes daily in a lapis gem elixir, charged by the light of a full moon for full vision.

365 Days of Health

Day 297:

"Eating sweets gives you no strength." -- Japanese Proverb

Day 298:

Any painful region may be cleansed and relieved by wearing a ring of iron near it regularly.

Day 299:

Blood gathered from a scratch at the back of your neck, and placed in a stream, will carry your maladies away with it.

Day 300:

Always pass the food at your table clockwise for health and luck. This is also true of beverages.

Day 301:

Bind your left hand to an apple tree with tri-colored yarn. Slip your hand out of the knot to leave any sickness or disease bound to the tree.

Day 302:

If your birth path number (add the month, date and year of your birth together; e.g. October 1, 1964 = 10+1+1+9+9+4 = 34 = 3+4 =7) is 6, you should take extra care with your health as this is a delicate matter in your life.

365 Days of Health

Day 303:

Sea vapor (dew) if gathered at dawn and applied to the skin promotes health. You can collect this by hanging out a natural cloth at sundown and wringing it out.

Day 304:

Washing one's body before the bells ring on Sunday eases any pain.

Day 305:

On All Saint's Day, gather 9 ivy leaves and put them under your pill. If you dream of improved health after this, your body will recover.

Day 306:

Ogam signs from the Celtic language may be inscribed on items to encourage well being. Here are a few:

⊢   Beth for purification and change

⪽   Saille to restore physical balance

⊣   Duir for strength

≢   Ur for healing

Day 307:

To safeguard your home from illness, place basil in all four corners of each room throughout the house. Make sure the herb is undisturbed or replace it with fresh on a regular basis.

Day 308:

Thought for the day: "To become a thoroughly good man is the best prescription for keeping a sound mind and a sound body." -- Francis Bowen

Day 309:

Take a thorn and place it against your side in a cloth for seven days. When you remove it, burn the thorn to likewise remove the thorn of sickness from your body.

Day 310:

To insure you get the proper rest essential for maintaining health, make a pillow stuffed with hops and balsam needles.

Day 311:

When everyone in your home seems to be getting sick, sweep the floors from the middle of the room toward the doors with a broom fashioned from a pine branch and dipped in rue tincture.

Day 312:

To make an incense to promote health and healing mix one teaspoon each of any of the following herbs (totaling 7 herbs) with one cup of sandalwood powder: carnation petals, powdered cinnamon, clove, lavender, myrrh, rose petals, rosemary, apple peel, hazel, orange rind, mint and/or savory.

365 Days of Health

Day 313:

Slice an apple crosswise to reveal a pentagram. Place this apple slice in cider and drink seven sips for well being. Dry and carry the slice as a health amulet.

365 Days of Health

Day 314:

To safeguard a newborn from illness, carry a flaming fir candle around its crib three times.

Day 315:

During Martinmas eat meat for health and to safeguard yourself from a sudden, untimely death.

Day 316:

Sprinkle healing herbs over a picture of a person who you know is ailing. Leave the herbs thereon to encourage recuperation. Once the person gets well, burn the herbs to dispel the sickness completely.

Day 317:

In Germany, runes were often inscribed on objects to produce specific magical energies, including those for health. Here are a few you can try:

þ   Inner Strength

<   Vitality

∫   End to troubles, change

↳   Turn arounds

Day 318:

Take a sword, dagger or good knife and in the air scribe the image of Thor's hammer over all the doorways and windows (an upside down capital T). This protects the home against sickness and disease.

Day 319:

Mugwort and daisy petals mixed with grease and applied to the back of the neck eases neck pain and stiffness.

Day 320:

To make a poultice for swelling mix warm barley mingled with fleawort, honey and lily oil.

Day 321:

If a remedial calls for wood bark, it should be gathered from the eastern side of a tree before noon for best results. East is the direction of the new day, a time of renewal and hope.

Day 322:

A woman who has recently given birth may safeguard her health by drinking a little of her mother's milk mixed with the juice of baked garlic.

Day 323:

To maintain strength and vitality, anoint yourself with cinnamon oil 2-3 times a week before bed time. Caution: some people are sensitive to this oil.

Day 324:

Saffron, red rose leaves, sandalwood, aloe and amber worn on one's head at night keeps sickness at bay.

365 Days of Health

Day 325:

Grape juice warmed with mulberry bark may be used to rinse one's mouth, thereby keeping teeth and gums healthy.

Day 326:

In Ceylon miniature swords sheathed in gold or silver are worn as health charms.

365 Days of Health

Day 327:

"The ingredients for health and long life are great temperance, open air, easy labor and little care."
-- Sir P. Sidney

Day 328:

Gather white rhubarb root at dawn and smash it. Place this in a square linen pouch and wear it to prevent cramps.

Day 329:

The festival honoring St. Catherine of Alexandra. To cure tumors, skin conditions and kidney stones, make a pilgrimage to a sacred well today and bathe therein.

Day 330:

To ease frostbite, Newfoundland healers recommend birch bark mingled with cod liver oil. When this same wood is used for broom handles, the tool can sweep away ill-health.

Day 331:

When a child is born the umbilical cord should be saved. Later in life this may be carried as a ward against disease.

Day 332:

Wear a crown of amaranth to promote longevity. In Greek, this flower's name means "never fading."

365 Days of Health

Day 333:

Nine shoots of ash root buried in a bottle will likewise bury sickness.

Day 334:

On Saint Andrews day the Scottish travel around their houses and towns with bells to drive out the malevolent spirits that cause sickness.

Day 335:

Put tansy in your shoe in winter to avoid colds and fever. This should be replaced regularly for effectiveness. Or, eat fist to internalize the energy of health.

Day 336:

Dill boiled in wine, then applied by a cloth to the nose will cure hiccough. Alternatively, try drinking fennel tea.

Day 337:

Knot grass gathered under a waning moon is a good amulet for health, especially for one's eye sight.

365 Days of Health

Day 338:

Thought for the day: "Keep yourself in health through exercise, and in heart through joyfulness."
-- Sir P. Sidney

365 Days of Health

Day 339:

Black, kidney-shaped pebbles are good all-purpose health amulets.

Day 340:

Peony root cut in square sections and worn is an effective charm to promote good health.

Day 341:

Placing a toad or a spider in a large nut shell will close sickness away from you. For a more humane alternative, use carvings.

Day 342:

Vervain gathered when the dog star rises and the sun and moon cannot be seen will protect the owner from all disease.

Day 343:

When folk remedials call for water, it is best taken from a south running stream.

Day 344:

Honey mixed with a pinch of salt and take from a seashell before dawn promotes health.

Day 345:

Wearing bells protects you against the spirits who bring sickness and disease. Additionally, they are very festive at this time of year!

Day 346:

Placing the fourth book of the Iliad under the pillow of an ailing person aids recovery.

Day 347:

"In these days half our diseases come from neglect of the body and overwork of the brain." -- Lytton Bulwer

Day 348:

In Sweden wearing a ring fashioned from mistletoe is considered both an effective cure and protection for one's health.

Day 349:

Hang an empty bottle in a chimney for seven days to collect all the sickness in the house. Cap it tightly at dusk, then destroy the bottle.

Day 350:

Placing peony flowers on an ailing person at noon will speed their return to health.

Day 351:

Pieces of cork connected with red silk ribbons and worn is effective to bind pain, especially cramps and stitches.

Day 352:

Bind a piece of your hair to a sturdy oak tree to give yourself more physical strength. If the tree ever seems to wither, remove the hair immediately.

365 Days of Health

Day 353:

Sacred words written and encased in green silk sewn in the form of a maltese cross bring the virtue of health to the bearer.

Day 354:

During the winter solstice, people in Japan eat pork dumplings at breakfast for continued health. Additionally, rice is fed to trees to encourage providence.

Day 355:

In all remedials the use of holy water will increase the effectiveness of the cure. Also, sprinkling it around one's house wards against disease.

Day 356:

Russians eat no meat until the first star appears on this day to insure their well being. Armenians eat fish, lettuce and spinach for similar purposes.

Day 357:

"Good medicine has often a bitter smack."
-- Japanese proverb

Day 358:

Save all the ashes from the Yule log tonight. Sprinkling these around your house will protect it from illness and storms. Also, don't let this log totally burn away as that is very bad luck.

Day 359:

According to Anglo Saxon tradition, each person in your household should stir the christmas pudding once clockwise while making a wish for health (or other wishes that might be important). This wish will come true on the New Year.

Day 360:

Giving your animals barley, oats and a little blessed salt today is said to encourage their health.

Day 361:

St. John's Day. Make small loaves of brown bread using holy wine to give all those who eat thereof immunity from poisons for 1 year. Additionally, all wine in the house should be blessed so those who drink it receive good health.

Day 362:

Thought for the day: "For every yuletide cake and every cheese tasted at a neighbor's house, a happy, healthy month will be added to one's life." -- Old English saying.

365 Days of Health

Day 363:

Place seven mullein leaves in your shoes today to prevent colds.

Day 364:

To alleviate pain, mingle mugwort, seven spoonfuls of moss, seven spoonfuls of ashes, milk and lard together and lay it on the region which hurts for seven minutes.

Day 365:

On New Year's eve, make a spiced red wine using cloves, a little brown sugar, orange slices, and cinnamon. This is called Waes Hael, which literally means "Be well!"

Postscript

This book has been set up by days instead of dates because many holidays and special observances shift from year to year depending on the day of the week. Consequently some entries might shift in their appropriateness from year to year.

Additionally, many of the ideas and suggestions found herein are timeless in appeal. This book is not carved in stone, so don't be afraid to get creative. Use Day 3's entry on Day 365 if you wish. After all, you are the Master of your Destiny, and life is, indeed, what we choose to make it. When more you take the reins of control back and dictate your own path, taking better care of yourself follows naturally. The end result is mentally, spiritually and physically fit living that comes from appreciating yourself and what you have, while striving to achieve your dreams.

Always reach for the stars with one foot on terra-firma and you will not be disappointed.

Heartily Yours,
Trish

More From Blue Star Productions

From the Hearts of Angels, Dezra*   12.95 U.S.
365 angels to guide you through any situation that may arise. Can be used for daily inspiration, finding your 'angel of the day,' or simply to find an answer to a problem.

Little Book of Angels, Dezra*   6.95 U.S.
Little Book of Angels Reflections Journal, Dezra*   5.95 U.S.
365 angels to provide a daily inspirational thought. The companion journal is perfect for recording your private responses to your angel's message.

The Antilles Incident, Todd   6.95 U.S.
A true face-to-face confrontation at sea with a submerged UFO.

365 Days of Prosperity, Telesco   5.95 U.S.
365 Days of Luck, Telesco   5.95 U.S.
365 Days of Health, Telesco   5.95 U.S.
Each of these little books contain daily ways to attract prosperity, luck, and health into your life!

Cataclysms?? A <u>New</u> Look at Earth Changes, Hickox   12.95 U.S.
A controversial approach to what some say are the coming 'end times.' This author claims messages picked up during the last 10 years are messages of past events, not coming attractions! Highly recommended.

The Ascent: Doorway to Eternity, Cross
  6. 95 U.S.
A channeled book regarding the true story of Jesus and his life as it was meant to be written. Truly enlightening!

To order, send check or money order, plus $3 s/h for one book, .50 for each additional book to: Book World, Inc., 9666 E Riggs Rd #194, Sun Lakes, AZ 85248.

Name: _____

Address: _____

City: _____

State: _____ Zip: _____